A GUIDE TO RUNNING YOUR FIRST MARATHON

DOUG LIMBRICK

This is the third revision of this guide — 2017.

Copyright© 2017 Doug Limbrick
All Rights Reserved

Cataloguing-in-Publication details available from the National Library of Australia.

ISBN: 978-0-646-97596-2

Cover design: Jeremy Limbrick

Typesetting/design and publishing assistance by
Publicious Book Publishing
www.publicious.com.au

The information contained in Appendix I of this publication may be copied in full or part by individuals to use as a training guide. However, the copying of Appendix I for other purposes or the copying of other parts of the publication will require the written permission of the author.

The author is an experienced marathon runner having completed 25 marathons with a PB of 2:57:05.

Other nonfiction publications by the author include:

Running the Marathon with Cancer. 2017

For information about other publications by the author: www.douglimbrick.com.

Comments and enquiries: info@douglimbrick.com

Note to readers about measurement:
The distances and other measures are provided in metric (e.g. metres, litres, etc) and the equivalent or near equivalent in imperial are provided in brackets.

Acknowledgements

I would like to thank those runners who provided feedback on earlier versions of this guide, which have been valuable in encouraging me to enhance and expand the information provided in this new version. I am extremely grateful to Jeremy Limbrick for the graphic design assistance he has provided including the cover design. Thanks also to my editor Dr Pam Faulks (Clarity Proofreading & Editing). I would also like to acknowledge that the McLachlan cartoon used in this guide is reproduced with permission of Punch Ltd., www.punch.co.uk.

*"If you want to run, run a mile.
If you want to experience another life,
run a marathon."*

Emil Zatopek[1]

---

[1] Emil Zátopek was a Czechoslovak long-distance runner best known for winning three gold medals at the 1952 Summer Olympics in Helsinki (5000 m, 10,000 m & the marathon).

Table of Contents

Introduction i
Who Can Run a Marathon? 1
How Much Time Do I Need to Prepare? 1
Commitment 5
The Long Run 6
Speed Work 12
Stretching and Exercises 15
Running Efficiently 17
Injuries 18
Food 21
Hydration 23
Running Gear 26
The Taper 28
Tactics 30
Marathon Weekend 31
Recovery 33
Appendix 1 – Marathon Training Program 38
Appendix 2 – Useful Stretches and Exercises 44
Some Further Reading 49

Introduction

There comes a time for many runners when the lure of running 42.2 kilometres (26 miles 385 yards) becomes difficult to resist. For some runners, this has been a long time in gestation and there is suddenly a need to do something about it, possibly a significant birthday is the trigger. I am aware of some runners who have it on their bucket list without any timeframe in mind, and others who suddenly decide they need a challenge and running a marathon becomes that challenge.

Whatever your reason, achieving the goal of running a marathon is possible for most people. It's a matter of committing yourself to undertaking the extra training that is required to conquer the marathon. That commitment will involve sticking to a program for a period of time and ensuring that the training becomes a priority. It's easy to commence a program and then start to skip sessions as time seems to drag on and you get tired. Understand that you will get tired and by the third month you may be wondering why you decided to train for a marathon. The idea behind marathon preparation is to ensure that you are very well prepared for the event and that when you eventually run the marathon, it seems relatively easy compared to the training program. Hence on race day you can do your best and enjoy the marathon atmosphere and the event.

I have been running for about 30 years. I have run in lots of events, including cross-country and mountain running, and have completed over 60 half marathons and 25 marathons. With the right training, I have managed a few sub three-hour finishes. It took me a little while to get the training and the race day strategy right to enable me to finish under three hours. I learnt much from experimenting with the quality, quantity and type of training that was required. I have been fortunate to have been asked to mentor a number of people to enable them to complete their first marathon.

This marathon guide is based on my own experiences of preparing to complete a number of marathons, and of assisting others to also achieve their goal of running a marathon. I trust there is some wisdom in what I have distilled from my experience and that it will enable you to achieve your goal. I believe that running 42.2 kilometres (26 miles 385 yards) is very different to any other event; it's a mental and emotional experience as well as a physical challenge. Be careful — it's addictive! Happy running.

Doug Limbrick.

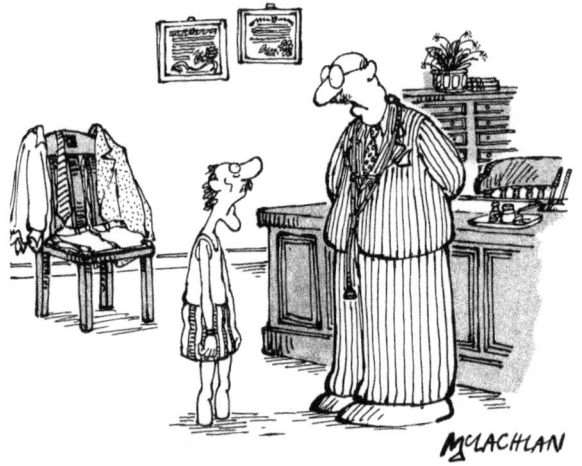

"Well, Mr Kerslake, I strongly recommend you give up marathon running." [2]

---

2. Reproduced with permission of Punch Ltd., www.punch.co.uk

Who Can Run a Marathon?

If you are a regular runner (i.e. you run several times a week) and have no medical or serious injury problems then, with additional training, there is no reason why you could not complete a marathon. If you have existing problems you should discuss your desire to run a marathon with your doctor or your sports medicine specialist. Your finish time will clearly relate to your current base level of fitness, the distances you are currently running, the frequency of your running, the amount of additional marathon training you do and, of course, your ability.

How Much Time Do I Need to Prepare?

Most marathon training programs are based on a 12-week program (although some are longer), followed by a two-week taper period immediately before the marathon. Thus, if you were preparing to run in an autumn marathon in the southern hemisphere in say April (an ideal time to run a marathon) you would train through January, February and March and use the first two weeks of April to taper. The 12-week program seems to be sufficient time for most runners to prepare provided that the existing base level of training is high enough (i.e. you are already running 4–5 times a week between 6 and 10 kilometres [4-6 miles] each time). If your base level is not high enough then don't commence the 12-week program until you have lifted your base level sufficiently.

The typical 12-week program involves a variety of hard and easy or recovery runs. For the first-time marathoner who already runs 4–5 times a week, a typical marathon-training week might consist of:

- **Monday:** medium run 10–12 kilometres (6-8 miles), starting the run at a comfortable training pace and gradually increasing the intensity to about the pace you will run the marathon. Your aim should be to run these at a faster pace than the weekly long run. You might gradually extend this run so that you are up to about 16 to 20 kilometres (10-12 miles) by the time you get to the third month.
- **Tuesday:** easy day 5–8 kilometres (3-5 miles).
- **Wednesday:** hard day with some speed work, involving tempo or intervals (see later explanation). This will help you run the marathon faster than would otherwise be the case. However, if you do not want to do any speed work then substitute another longer run similar to Monday.
- **Thursday:** easy day 5–8 kilometres (3-5 miles).

- **Friday:** easy day 5–8 kilometres (3-5 miles).
- **Saturday:** hard day involving the long run for the week. Depending on your level of fitness you might start in week one with a run of 15–20 kilometres (9-12 miles) and increase the distance by about 10% each week. The aim is to progressively move to long runs of around 28–34 kilometres (17-21 miles) or, more importantly, be able to run for 3–3.5 hours (without worrying about your pace or the distance covered). This is the most important run in the program for the first-time marathoner. The more of these you can complete the better prepared you will be to face the 42.2 kilometres (26 miles 385 yards) on marathon day (see later section on the long run).
- **Sunday:** easy day or rest day. Some runners include a rest day in their marathon-training program and generally do this after the long run as a recovery day. If you have difficulty taking a day off you might consider cross training on that day e.g. cycling or swimming. However, if you do run be sure to have an easy short run (3–5 kilometres; 2-3 miles) to get the stiffness out of your legs from the long run (include 2–3 short stride outs at a quicker pace).

This of course is only one example of how a marathon-training program might be structured. You could take this mix of runs and completely change the sequence to suit your requirements. You might want to include two speed sessions per week, or you might like more time to recover between your long run and your medium-length run. Some people prefer to do their long run on Sundays and hence will structure the week a little differently to the above program. Flexibility is fine, but it is essential for you to complete a number of the long runs if you are to succeed in your quest to run a marathon. Appendix 1 contains greater detail on how to structure a three-month marathon-training program.

If your training is interrupted and you miss a long run or need to take a day or so off running because of a minor injury or some personal event then don't be concerned. Similarly, if you have a bad long run don't be concerned. The program is a three-month program and you are seeking to benefit from the total program and not one single component. Simply resume your program when you are able and don't try to make up for the lost runs.

Commitment

Before launching further into the program it's necessary to talk about commitment. One of the hardest things about preparing for a marathon is sticking to the program. A key reason that runners don't get to the start line or don't finish a marathon is lack of commitment to the program. If you are serious about doing a marathon, then you have to be serious about sticking to the program. The first month will pass fairly quickly, but as time goes on you will start to feel tired from the extra distance and you may start to have doubts about the wisdom of continuing the program. There will also be a few extra aches and you may question your ability to run a marathon. Don't worry, these thoughts are normal. Commit to the program and stick to it and you will run a marathon. As I indicated above, it's a three-month program and so its okay to miss a run or two if you are extra tired or have an injury or are feeling unwell, but not if something more exciting comes up. Once you start missing sessions for reasons other than tiredness, illness or injury then the program will soon disintegrate. The cornerstone of the program is the long run, so try not to miss these unless you think it unwise to proceed. If you listen to your body you will know if you need a rest. Remember that tiredness and a few aches and pains are a normal consequence of preparing for a marathon.

The Long Run

The long run is designed to:
- prepare you mentally for the marathon (you will know what it's like to run for a long time and to keep running when your legs are tired and sore)
- give you strength and endurance and thus prepare you physically for the marathon
- prepare your body to be able to store more glycogen than would otherwise be the case
- enable you to practice doing what you will do during the marathon, such as drinking on the run.

The question usually asked by the first-time marathoner is how long should my first long run be. Clearly this will depend on your current level of training. If you are already doing a 12–15 kilometre (7-9 mile) run each week then you may be able to start with an 18–20 kilometre (11-12 mile) run as your first long run. The aim is to move towards the 30 kilometre (18 mile) mark by the end of your first month of training. It's okay to walk during this long run if you need to. However, your aim should be to get to a point where you can run the total distance during your long run. A guide is that this run should occupy about 20–30 per cent of your weekly distance. I ran my first marathon (when I was much younger) with five long runs: two at 25 kilometres (15 miles) and three at 27 kilometres (17 miles) and finished in 3:18 — a couple of minutes inside my desired finish time. However, I subsequently discovered that by increasing the distance of my long runs to over 30 kilometres (18 miles) I finished faster and much stronger.

I have been asked many times two questions about the long run:
- Ideally, how far should the longest run be?
- Should I run a slow full marathon before the event?

The answer to the second question is definitely no — you should not attempt to run the full distance before the event. Firstly, it's unnecessary and, secondly, it may prevent you from participating in the event. Running that distance will leave you feeling depleted and you will need to take time off from your training to recover, and you may injure yourself and not get to run the marathon. That gets us back to the first question. You should aim to do a few runs of over 30 kilometres (18 miles). It would be good if one or two of those runs were 34 or 35 kilometres (21-22 miles). There is no precise rule about this. Clearly, if you do the work for three months then you should finish without having to walk, provided that you run sensibly on the day (e.g. don't start too fast). However, it is clear that the more long runs you are able to complete as part of your preparation, the better prepared you will be, the more confident you will be, and you should experience less discomfort in the last 10 kilometres (6 miles) or so.

Another way to look at your long run is to appreciate that one of its key functions is to equip you to stay on your feet for a long period of time. Thus, some marathoners declare that the distance of the long run is not important and the aim is to progressively increase the duration of the run. Hence the first long run might be 1.5 hours with an increase in time each week. The longer you predict you will take to run a marathon, the longer in time (not distance) should be your long run. It's difficult to be more specific, but as a guide:
- If you will take upwards of 4 hours, then you should have at least one run of about 3.5 hours.
- If you are an intermediate marathoner in the range of 3.25 to 3.75 hours, then a few runs around the 3-hour mark will be helpful,
- If you are an elite level runner, then your long runs may not need to be over 2.5 hours.

It's also important to remember that speed is not important on the long run (use your mid-week run for speed training). Run easy and relaxed for the first part of the run and gradually pick up the pace. It's fine to run these at 30–60 seconds per kilometre (45-90 seconds per mile) slower than you intend to run the marathon. This is not a speed session.

It's useful to try and do your long runs with at least one other person. It helps with motivation and the time also seems to pass more quickly. Try to find a training partner or a group you can join. Enquire at your local running club and you will usually find that there are people training for a marathon that you can join and there may also be structured training programs.

Ideally, you should aim to do your last long run two weeks before the marathon. This will ensure that you recover fully before the marathon and remember that long runs done after this point will not improve your performance. In fact, it is okay to start your taper three weeks out from the marathon if you have completed a number of long runs. However, most experienced marathon runners will do a long run of 30 kilometres (18 miles) or more two weeks before the event. For the first timer it's best to recover well from your hard work in the previous weeks and thus on the weekend two weeks from the event it would be fine to do a moderate length run of say 18–20 kilometres (11-12 miles) rather than a run of over 30 kilometres (18 miles).

If you are doing your long runs on a softer type surface, such as you might encounter if running a forest trail, then it is a good idea to do at least one of the long runs on bitumen. While the trails are great to run on and may involve less soreness in your legs after a long run they don't represent the surface you will run on during the event. In most marathons you will be running on bitumen, which is more demanding on your legs. Hence, you need to run at least one of the 30+ kilometre (18+ mile) runs on bitumen (possibly the last one).

A word of warning about possible chafing during the long run. You will perspire on the long runs and you and your running clothes may become saturated. This often leads to chafing. The most common places are the inner thighs where your shorts may rub when wet, the underarm area where your singlet or T-shirt may rub and, particularly for men, the nipples where the wet singlet or T-shirt rubs (bleeding nipples are very painful). Most marathon runners use either Vaseline (petroleum jelly) or one of the commercial products designed specifically for this purpose (often applied from a roll-on or stick and sometimes used by swimmers and triathletes to facilitate use of a wetsuit). Some runners tape these areas. I have always used Vaseline and have never had a chafing problem during a marathon. You will need to experiment to determine which method suits you best. It's extremely important to prevent chafing as a bad case of chafing could prevent you from finishing a marathon.

If you are like me, you will choose to do your long run first thing in the morning, which is clearly a good idea if you are training through the summer period. It also means that the long run becomes your first priority for the day and so it's not left to later in the day when events may occur that could prevent you from undertaking the run. Doing the run early does raise the question of eating before the run. You have just had a good sleep and your last meal was probably your dinner last night. Now you are about to run 30 kilometres (18 miles) or so. Assuming that you have loaded up with lots of carbohydrates and some protein at that meal, then you will have stored fuel. Some people are capable of eating breakfast before the long run without any problems during that run, but most people can't do that as they will be very uncomfortable and will probably get a stitch, which if severe enough may terminate the run. I have found that I need to eat something before the run so that I am not running with an empty stomach and I find that a small mount of extra fuel is useful to ensuring a good run takes place. I experimented and found that if I consumed a small amount of food (with some water or sports drink) it did not cause any problems. I started with a savoury biscuit with honey before my first long run and slightly increased the amount with each run so that by about the 4th or 5th long run I could eat a piece of toast with honey or half a banana. This provided some extra fuel and took away that empty feeling. I was then able to supplement the fuel by consuming some gels along the way.

Speed Work

As I indicated earlier, this component is not mandatory (unlike the long run). However, speed work will benefit you in several ways as it will:
- enable a quicker finish time
- aid you in finishing because it contributes to endurance
- give you added confidence that you have prepared well
- help break up your training and make it

more interesting, exposing you to a different type of training experience.

Elite and experienced athletes will do fast workouts at least twice a week. The first-time and non-elite marathoner should definitely consider including a weekly session in their program. Fast workouts are generally of two types: repeats/intervals and tempo runs.

Repeats/intervals involve running fast (at a pace around your 5–10 kilometres or 3-6 miles race pace) for a given distance (200–1500 metres or 220-1640 yards) and repeating this several times (repeats) with a recovery (interval) between each one. These repeats are often done on a track or oval where the distance around is known. For marathon training maximum benefit will come from doing longer distance repeats e.g. 800, 1200 and 1500 metres (880, 1320 and 1650 yards). The recovery interval should be long enough to enable your heart rate to come back to where it was before the repeat. After some practice, you may only need a 200-metre (220 yard) recovery interval. Always move (walk or jog slowly) during the interval as if you stop you will dramatically reduce the benefit of the session. The aim is to be able to do the repeats at an even pace so that the pace of the first one is the same as the pace for the last one. If you are slowing down then you are running too fast during the early repeats. Start with some 200 and 400 metre (220 and 440 yard) repeats and work up to the longer distances. For example, you might aim to be able to do a session by the mid-point in the three-month program comprising a 400, 800, 1200, 800, 400 (440, 880, 1320, 880, 440 yards) with a 200 (220 yard) recovery between each one.

Ensure that you warm up and cool down with a 10–15 minute easy run before and after each session. You might ideally run slowly to the oval, do your speed work, and then run slowly home.

Tempo runs are not as intense as the long repeats but they help with speed and enable you to run faster during the marathon without producing debilitating amounts of lactic acid. You run these at 10–15 seconds a kilometre (20-30 seconds a mile) slower than your 10-kilometre (6 mile) race pace. Warm up and cool down with an easy run of 2–3 kilometres (1-2 miles). You can do a continuous single tempo run or a set. The continuous run could involve a 10-minute warm up, 20-minute tempo and 10-minute cool down. After a month to six weeks of training you might be able to do a set comprising four to six 1-kilometre (0.6 mile) repeats at tempo pace with a 60 seconds recovery jog between each one.

You might like to do repeats one week and tempo work the next. Another way of adding some faster work is to participate in some fun runs or club runs of 5–10 kilometres (3-6 miles) and push yourself so that you are running faster than your normal training runs. Most clubs have weekly runs and are happy for non-members to participate by paying a small entry fee (if you do a few of these it may be cheaper to join as most clubs have a relatively inexpensive annual fee).

Stretching and Exercises

The consensus among regular runners is that stretching before and after a run is useful in reducing stiffness, minimising injury, assisting recovery and increasing suppleness. While some runners skip the pre-run stretching I believe that a brief stretching session before a run will help you prepare mentally for the run and will contribute to the warm up. This session should not be too vigorous. For example, gently stretch the hamstrings, the quads and the muscles in the lower part of the legs. The session after a run can be much more vigorous and extensive because the muscles are warm and much more flexible. While you can stretch further and longer after a run ensure that the stretch is smooth (not jerky) and is done to the point where you can feel the stretch occurring (it should not be painful). Hold each stretch for about 30 seconds. I have included the basic stretches in Appendix 2.

If you are competing in races as a part of your training then be sure to undertake a cool down run after the race. This will help avoid stiffness. It's also useful if you can stand in cold water (a stream or a lake or the bath) after your long run, as this will aid recovery. The elite runners often use an ice bath to promote recovery.

There are many other stretches and exercises that will assist you to run more smoothly and avoid injury. While your main aim is to stick to the marathon program there are some basic exercises that won't take much time and will add to your marathon preparation. For example, strengthening your core will help in a number of ways. Possibly the most effective core exercise is the plank (see Appendix 2). Doing a core exercise three to four times a week will assist your overall fitness. However, don't get carried away by adding lots of new exercises as you could injure yourself and miss the marathon. If you do add new exercises be sure to do so early in the program. Remember that your main focus should be on the basic marathon program.

Running Efficiently

We all have different running styles. Some runners look smooth while others look awkward and off balance while running. No matter what our running style is we all get there sooner or later. However, it's worth contemplating running styles when considering running efficiency and distance running. Once you move up to the marathon distance efficiency becomes more important because it's linked to conserving energy, which is of course very useful for a marathoner. There are a couple of useful things to consider that may make running 42.2 kilometres (26 miles 385 yards) a little bit easier.

Firstly, it's useful to look at your stride. Do you take big steps? Stride- outs are useful over a very small distance to help with stiffness but are not for marathon running. Big strides are for sprinters. If you have ever watched elite marathon runners you will have observed that they take small strides almost like a shuffle. That's because it's the most efficient way to run long distances. Hence it's worth checking your stride to see if you need to modify it (don't be concerned if you try and it doesn't work for you). Sports scientists have done some work on this subject and have concluded that shortening your stride can reduce injury. It seems that a reduction of 5 to 10 per cent puts less strain on areas that are frequently injured when training intensity is increased, such as IT bands and knees. The shorter stride involves less impact.

The second thing that may increase your efficiency is to look at your arm swing. You will notice that sprinters have a very exaggerated arm movement like a pumping action. As a marathon runner its best to have short arm movements as this conserves energy. It's also important to ensure that your arms move back and forward in a straight line. Some runners move their arms across their body, which results in shoulder movement. This has the effect of pulling you off balance (it appears to be a style more common with women). Eliminating the arm movement across the body and the shoulder movement can increase efficiency and conserve energy. If you find that you run like this its worth trying to modify it but don't become obsessed with it. If you can't correct your arm swing then that's okay you will still get to the finish even if a little less efficiently.

Injuries

Given your increased training distances and intensity you will be at greater risk of sustaining an injury. It is important to try as much as possible to maintain a preventative strategy during your training program. This will rely on you managing your program in a sensible manner. Be sure that you:

- don't increase your distance or intensity dramatically (10 per cent increases are manageable)
- don't have two hard training days in a row (or if you do ensure that you follow with two easy days)
- listen to your body, it will tell you if you need to pull back or rest
- stretch properly and cool down
- eat and drink adequately to match your level of training
- get enough rest (you will most certainly need more sleep during this training period)
- wear good shoes suitable for distance running and for your biomechanics (don't rely on your old faithfuls – in fact, it's best to have two pairs of shoes because it's been demonstrated that alternating shoes reduces the possibility of certain types of injuries)
- if you are a beginner runner stay away from hills until you build leg-muscle strength (once you have good leg strength then hill running once or twice a week will further strengthen your legs against injury)

- be sensible regarding the intensity of any speed work you do. For example, run your current 5-kilometre (3 mile) race pace for intervals of 1200 metres (1320 yards) or less, and your current 10-kilometre (6 mile) pace for longer intervals.

All runners experience aches and soreness during marathon training. This is largely due to some damage to the muscles. Remember that each time the exercise is performed the damage is a little less. The best strategy to avoid muscle soreness is to use the muscles again and again. In most instances aches and soreness from the increased training can be managed with ice, massage, stretching, elevation and rest. If soreness develops don't ignore it. Its best to treat it aggressively by applying ice to the affected area and keeping it elevated if appropriate. However, if you do become injured seek assistance from a sports medicine specialist as soon as possible. You will need to determine if the problem is more than soreness due to increased training. If the pain is uncharacteristically intense and persistent the chances are that its more than some muscle damage and will need correct diagnosis and treatment. A sports medicine specialist will work with you to keep you going with your training if at all possible.

Don't worry about sore and black toenails. This happens to most distance runners. You may lose a toenail before your training is complete.

Let me emphasise that the most important preventative strategy that you can adopt as a runner — particularly as a distance runner — is to develop the habit of listening to your body. The signals that you get from your body will enable you to modify or change your training so as to prevent an injury that may end your chances of achieving your goal of running a marathon.

Food

As you increase your marathon training you are likely to feel hungry more often. It's best to respond to this with an increase in the foods that will provide the power for your runs. Carbohydrates are the foods that will translate into energy. Both simple and complex carbohydrates are useful as a source of marathon food. However, it's more important to eat plenty of complex carbohydrates (e.g. fruit, vegetables, pasta and rice). While the focus for a marathoner is on the carbohydrates for fuel it is important to ensure that you maintain a balanced diet (don't neglect protein intake by substituting more carbohydrate for your normal protein intake).

The increased training will place your body under increased stress, particularly after your long run. Hence the balanced diet is very important to keeping you healthy. Eat as soon as you can after your hard runs, particularly the long run, as this will speed recovery (eating something within half an hour is very important). The sooner you eat the more effective it will be in aiding the recovery process. Try a banana or a sports bar.

You may need to experiment a little to find the carbohydrates that suit your body best and the overall diet that works for you. If you do experiment with different foods do it in the early part of your training in order to settle into a good food routine as early as possible. Dramatic changes to food intake close to the marathon could be disastrous. If possible, in the two days before the marathon increase the amount of carbohydrate in your diet (possibly decrease the amount of fibre as you don't want to upset the system). It's important to ensure that you are not hungry during this period so that you don't deplete glycogen stores. It's also very important to be well hydrated at this time, as you cannot build up your glycogen reserves if you are not properly hydrated.

Eating food during the marathon is generally not possible for most marathoners. If you intend to eat then you need to practice this during your training to ensure that it does not upset your system or cause a stitch. A much better way of taking energy in during the marathon is to ingest a sports gel about every 45 minutes. These gels replace electrolytes and salts and contain some carbohydrate (some also contain caffeine). However, you will need to practice this in order to get the technique right and to find the gel (brand, flavour, texture, etc.) that suits you best. You need to take these with some water or sports drink so that they move quickly from your stomach and are absorbed.

Hydration

It's very important to drink regularly in the period leading up to the marathon and during the running of the marathon. Dehydration during your training will prevent you from performing well and even mild dehydration could cause you to abort a training run. It is essential that you drink regularly during the marathon. Drink stations will usually be located at 5-kilometre (3 mile) intervals. Be sure to drink at each drink station. Don't miss the first drink station because you are not feeling thirsty. If you wait until you feel thirsty you are likely to already be dehydrated. You need this liquid on board early when your body can process and use it. Your stomach gradually shuts down as blood is moved away from that area to the outside of your body to keep you cool. Remember that at best your body can only replace a proportion of the liquid that is lost during extended periods of exercise. Continue to rehydrate after the exercise has finished.

Be sure to practice drinking during your long run by taking a water bottle along. Some marathon runners prefer water, others a sports drink and some mix their own special drink. There is evidence supporting the use of sports drinks during a marathon to replace the electrolytes and salts that are lost. The loss of these can result in muscle problems, which will progressively slow you down. You may also experience nausea and dizziness due to loss of electrolytes and salts.

The loss of sodium during endurance sports can cause a condition known as hyponatremia. Sodium is an electrolyte and helps regulate the amount of water that's in and around your cells. Drinking too much water may cause the remaining sodium in your body to become diluted. The condition has been referred to as "water intoxication". The symptoms of mild hyponatremia may include lethargy, headache, nausea and malaise. I experienced mild hyponatremia during a marathon and it cost me a sub- three-hour finish. I was running strongly when I went through the 32-kilometre (19 mile) mark and felt as though I would easily finish under 3 hours. Only 10 kilometres (6 miles) to go and I was feeling so good. Within a short time I started to feel nauseas and light headed and the nausea and light-headedness progressively increased in intensity over the remaining distance. I also felt tired in the legs and had to work extremely hard to keep running. I shuffled into the stadium and finished in 3:16.46. I had consumed only water and took on board more than usual because it was a relatively hot day. Since that experience I have only consumed sports drink and used the water to tip over myself.

If you have difficulty using sports drinks then it might be wise to alternate between water and sports drink from drink station to drink station. Experiment with different drinks and strengths to find what suits you best. Some marathons permit all runners (not just the elite runners) to have their special mixture placed at each drink station. It has been estimated that using a sports drink during a marathon can reduce your finish time by about 2 per cent.

Running Gear

The most important component of your gear is your shoes. You may be accustomed to running in inexpensive shoes but when you step up to marathon distance running it's important to have good fitting, comfortable and supportive shoes. You need a pair of shoes made for distance work. Purchase them early in your training and use them for your long run. Don't try to break in a new pair of shoes the week before the marathon. If you can afford two pair of shoes then you might get a less expensive but good pair of training shoes to complement your number one pair. Don't run in the same pair of shoes on consecutive days. This will help to avoid injury and your shoes will last longer (if allowed to dry between runs) and hold their shape better. Make sure that you use your running shoes exclusively for running. Using them for walking or other recreation purposes will decrease their value as running shoes.

There are many good brands of distance training shoes. Be sure to purchase your shoes from a specialist running shoe shop where those serving you are experienced runners. Take your time in selecting the shoes, try many pairs on and be sure that they fit you securely, but allow for expansion of your feet on those long runs (you will need approximately half a size more). There will be a running shoe that matches your height, weight, biomechanics etc., so take time to find it. Talk to the shop assistants about different lacing methods to find the one that holds your foot securely (particularly your heel) and suits you best.

If you wear socks then it would be worth investing in a couple of pairs of expensive running socks as they provide a greater degree of cushioning. Keep them exclusively for running and they will last for a long time.

The other items of your gear will largely be a matter of personal preference. Be sure to use the gear you intend to use during the marathon on your long runs so that it is well worn in and you have discovered any problems. Cotton gear, particularly shorts, may not be a wise choice because the cotton will absorb and hold moisture much more than synthetic material. During the marathon you will perspire and may tip cups of water over yourself to keep cool. Cotton shorts will become very heavy and may be more inclined to cause chafing. However, some runners still prefer cotton. Experiment with your top and shorts to achieve what will be best on marathon day. A minor problem during your training can become a major annoyance during those last 10 kilometres (6 miles) of the marathon. Eliminate these problems, no matter how small, before the marathon.

The Taper

It's very important that you reduce the intensity and quantity of your training in the two-week period immediately before the marathon and for the novice marathoner it may be best to start the taper three weeks before the event. You need to recover from all the additional training over the past three months and be fresh on marathon day. This will require a dramatic reduction in the level of your training during those two to three weeks. Once you get to that point in the program you have done all the hard work, you can now coast along till the marathon. Your longest run two weeks out should not be more than about 20 kilometres (12 miles). Discontinue the speed work during this period and progressively reduce your distances down to about 5–8 kilometres (3-5 miles) per day in the last week. You may find difficulty in cutting back during this taper period given the large amount of training you have done over the past three months. However, it's important that you recover fully by marathon day so you will have to be disciplined. Don't worry about losing your fitness. No amount of additional work during this period will help your performance. In fact, it will detract from it, may lead to an injury so close to the marathon and will leave you tired. Be careful not to overeat during this period. You have cut back on your training and should therefore not need the same level of fuel. The exception is during the two days before the marathon when you should try to overload with liquid and carbohydrate. The additional liquid helps keep you hydrated and "washes" the carbohydrate into the muscle tissues. Many marathon runners do a harder run of 7–15 kilometres (4-9 miles) at around marathon pace on the Wednesday before the marathon and then carbohydrate load through to the marathon.

Some experts advocate a no alcohol policy the week before a marathon. Alcohol collects in the muscle tissue, takes time to move on and has an impact on performance. Certainly, if you are looking for every possible way to enhance your performance then it would be wise to consider abstinence during the two days prior to the marathon (it takes about two days for alcohol to be cleared from the muscle tissues).

Tactics

Whatever you decide about your projected finish time or the splits you will run, be sure not to start too quickly. Remember this is not a 5, 10 or even 20-kilometre (3, 6 or 12 mile) race — it's a marathon of 42.2-kilometres (26 miles 385 yards). Don't get carried away at the start and run the first few kilometres (miles) too quickly or you will pay dearly in the latter part of the event. A fast start could result in you hitting the wall and not finishing. You will burn up precious glycogen with a fast start. It is not possible in a marathon to recover from a start that is faster than your training and ability permits. It is much better to start slowly and run the first few kilometres (miles) less quickly than you are capable of doing. This will assist you to finish running when others are walking. Marathon running is more a test of survival than competition. For most marathoners, the best way to run your best time is to run as even a pace as possible. Work out your projected finish time and then do your maths to determine how long it should take you to run each 5-kilometre (3 mile) split. This is your game plan. Be sure to stick to it and run each 5 kilometres (3 miles) at the same pace. For example, if you are a strong runner with a projected finish time of 3.30, then you should aim to run each kilometre in 4:58 (8 per mile) or 24:53 for each 5-kilometre (3 mile) split. The 4-hour finisher should aim for a time of 5:42 per kilometre (9.10 per mile) or 28:26 per 5-kilometre (3 mile) split.

Marathon Weekend

You have done the training and now the time has come for you to enjoy the event. If possible on marathon weekend mingle with the other runners. If there is a marathon expo attend it and soak up the atmosphere.

On the day before the marathon make sure you remain well hydrated. Drink small amounts often. It's best to drink a sports drink because the salts will work to help you maximise the level of hydration. They have the effect of slowing down the drainage from the stomach and so increase the amount absorbed into the body. If you drink only water you will be making regular trips to the toilet. Eat lots of carbohydrate and try not to eat any foods that may upset your system. In other words, it's not the time to try new foods - instead, concentrate on those you have used during your training. It's also wise to munch on carbohydrates during the day as you drink (try a banana, a sports bar or even some jelly babies).

The day before the marathon go for a slow 2–3 kilometre (1-2 mile) run and include in it some surges and strides over 20–30 metres (25-35 yards) at race pace (i.e. simply stride out for a short distance at your marathon pace). The purpose of this session is to eliminate any aches or strains, so that you do not carry them into the marathon. Finish with some good stretches of the major muscle groups.

Don't be concerned if you don't sleep well the night before the marathon (this is common, especially for first timers). If this happens your system will cope and it will not affect your performance. However, it is important to try to get a good night's sleep two nights prior to the marathon.

On marathon day be sure to rise in time to have a good breakfast before the marathon. This should take place at least three hours before start time. This is your last opportunity to fuel up before the marathon. Don't miss it.

Apply Vaseline or one of the body glide preparations strategically to ensure that you avoid chafing during the marathon. You should be familiar with this from your long runs.

About 10–15 minutes before the start of the marathon have a last pre-marathon drink. This will prime your stomach ready to receive and empty more fluid on the run to ensure that you remain hydrated during the marathon. You should consume about 5 ml per kilogram (2.2 pounds) of body weight. Hence a 65–kilogram (143 pounds) runner would need about 325 ml (11 oz) 10–15 minutes before the start. This might seem like a rather a large amount and therefore you need to practice this before each long run.

Stretch gently and jog slowly to the start. Place yourself appropriately in the pack (be modest). You are now ready to go. When the gun goes off remember your game plan and don't get carried away. Best of luck with your first marathon.

Recovery

Congratulations, you have completed your first marathon! Having achieved this you will be on a high for some time (although you may not have felt like that in the last few kilometres of the event). In the first couple of days after the event you will be tired, stiff and sore. Climbing or descending steps will be a challenge. Nevertheless, you will probably be looking forward to putting on your well-earned marathon T-shirt and going for a run as soon as possible. Don't! Your legs will feel tired and flat and you will be disappointed. Take time to recover properly. Bask in the glory of your triumph, bore you family and work colleagues with your marathon story and show them the pictures. Running the marathon has damaged some of your leg muscles and they need time to heal. If you must exercise soon after the marathon then cycle, swim or take a walk. The recovery process is different for each of us and so the recovery period will vary from person to person. Starting back too soon could mean that you feel flat for months. Whereas a reasonable period of rest and healing could have you back competing at your pre-marathon level almost as soon as you start back running. After my first couple of marathons I ran within 3–4 days and found I didn't enjoy the experience. I also felt flat during my running for weeks. Subsequently I experimented with the recovery process and I now take a 10-day rest from running after a marathon. In the first 5–7 days I do almost nothing except for some walking and then I cycle a little. I find that by doing this I am back to my normal race speeds very quickly.

My experience is supported by tests that have been done to compare marathon runners who ran in the week following the marathon and those who did no running in that week. Both groups were tested just after the event and endurance had dropped in both groups. However, by the third day after the marathon the non-running group's muscles began to improve while there was no improvement for running group. For the remainder of the week the non-running group scored consistently higher in tests on muscle strength and endurance. Neither group had any muscle soreness by day five yet the running group's leg muscles had clearly not recovered to the same extent as the non-running group. It was concluded that even when muscles feel okay they are unlikely to be functioning normally and be ready for regular exercise.

I mentioned above that running a marathon has caused damage to your leg muscles, which is the cause of post-marathon soreness. A little more information may assist you to decide when you should start to run again. Each of our muscles consists of many tiny fibres known as microfibres, which are bunched together. They are activated by nerves causing them to contract at the same time, resulting in the whole muscle contracting. Each contraction of these tiny microfibres can damage the cell wall (this occurs many times during a marathon). If the muscles were viewed under a microscope after a marathon they would show extensive tears to most microfibres. Each of these tears known as a micro-tear is damage that needs to heal. Within about 12 hours the damaged muscles swell as a result of an increase in white blood cells. Immune cells are also attracted and they cause further swelling and they release chemicals that cause pain. This is the pain that is felt during exercise recovery.

My advice therefore is that you take time to recover well and then start to plan your second marathon.

I have been asked by some first-time marathoners, buoyed by their recent success, how long they should wait until they run another marathon. This will clearly depend on how quickly you recover and how soon your body is able to cope with another marathon training program without injury problems arising. However, it is possible to back up and run another marathon fairly soon after your first marathon if you are sure that you have recovered sufficiently. I have run a second marathon a few times within a three-month period. My approach involved 10 days of no running (only some cycling and walking) and then some short runs each day for a week (8–10 kilometre or 5-6 miles) taking it easy on the flat. At the end of two weeks of running I did a 20-kilometre (12 miles) run to test my recovery and to see if I had retained the marathon fitness in my legs from the recent marathon. If that run went well I then stepped up the weekly long runs and moved back into the marathon-training program. However, if you contemplate doing your second marathon soon after your first one then be cautious as an injury could stop you from running for some time. I know from experience as I tried to move back into marathon training too soon after a marathon and damaged a hamstring (six weeks of no running was the result).

Marathon running is different from shorter distance running. Listen to your body and have a long marathon career.

Appendix 1 – Marathon Training Program

Clearly the intensity of this program at the start will depend on your current base level of fitness, the number of times you are running each week and your weekly total distance.

First month

Use this month to gradually increase the total distance each week, the distance of your shorter runs, introduce a long run and increase its length each week and start doing some speed work. By the end of the month you should be running a total weekly distance of 60 to 70 kilometres (36-42 miles).

Monday: Start with 8 kilometres (5 miles) and build up distance to 12 kilometres (8 miles) by the end of the month. This is one of your harder runs but do it on a flat course.
Tuesday: An easy run of 5 to 8 kilometres (3-5 miles).
Wednesday: Start doing speed work by introducing a tempo run each week. Do a 2-kilometre (1.25 miles) warm up and then run faster (a little slower than your 10-kilometre – 6 mile - race pace) for 250 metres (275 yards), then recover by running

slowly, then do another 250 metres (275 yards) fast, and then finish with a 2-kilometre (1.25 miles) warm down. Over the month increase the number of tempos or the distance of each one (e.g. 3 x 250 metres or 2 x 400 metres – 3 x 275 yards or 2 x 440 yards).

Thursday: If you are tired from your fast work have a rest day or do an easy 5 kilometres (3 miles).

Friday: This is an easy day before your long run so relax and run slowly but evenly for 5–8 kilometres (3-5 miles).

Saturday: This is the most important run of the week for marathon training. For example, start with 15–16 kilometres (9-10 miles) and increase the distance each week — 18–19 kilometres (11-12 miles), 21–22 kilometres (13-14 miles), 24–25 kilometres (15-16 miles). Your existing base may of course be sufficient to allow you to move the distance of your long run closer to 30 kilometres (18 miles) by the end of the month. Be sure to run these longer runs at a pace slower than your proposed marathon race pace (theses runs are referred to as LSD – long slow distance – runs).

Sunday: This can be a rest day or a day for cross training. Ensure that you use it to recover from the long run.

Second and third months

The program for each of these two months should be very similar.

Monday: Increase the length of this run a little 12–14 kilometres (8-10 miles) and introduce a hill or two but be sure to run at an easy pace.

Tuesday: An easy 8–9 kilometres (5-6 miles).

Wednesday: Alternate between tempo running one week and intervals the next week. Be sure to do a warm up and warm down run for each type of speed work. For the tempo runs increase the distance of your tempo component (500 metres to 1 kilometre – 500 to 1000 yards), with a 1–2 minutes recovery between each one. Do your intervals on an oval or track and start with some 200–250 metre (220-250 yards) fast bursts at your 5-kilometre (3 mile) race pace with a recovery between each one (say 100–200 metres – 110-220 yards). Be sure to run the fast components of your tempo and interval training at an even pace so that the speed of the first one is the same as the speed of your last one. If you find that you are slowing down then you are running the early ones too fast.

Thursday: An easy 5–6 kilometres (3-4 miles) or a rest day if you need it.

Friday: An easy run at an even pace of 8–10 kilometres (5-6 miles).

Saturday: Continue with your weekly long run at an easy pace (could be run at 1 minute slower than your proposed marathon race pace). Move to 28 kilometres (17 miles) as soon as possible, then to 30 kilometres (18 miles) and aim to do three to four runs of 33–34 kilometres (20-21 miles) before you start the taper (possibly even do one at 35 kilometres – 22 miles - if the training permits).

Sunday: A rest day is possibly a good idea for Sundays in these two months. You need to recover. If you must exercise then cycle or swim but ensure that these are easy sessions.

If you enter a race, say 5 or 10 kilometres (3-6 miles), during the three months program then run hard and substitute this for one of your hard days. It's not a good idea to do two hard days consecutively. This could easily lead to an injury.

The Taper

It's now time to concentrate on getting rid of those aches, pains and niggles before race day. In the next two (or three if you have decided on a longer taper) weeks you need to reduce the workload considerably. To do this you remove the hills, the speed work and the very long runs from the program. Your focus should be on easy running.

Your first taper week could involve a 10-kilometre (6 mile) run on Monday and Wednesday, with 5-kilometre (3 mile) runs on the other weekdays except on Saturday, when you might do 18–20 kilometres – 11-12 miles (this will be your last longish run before the marathon). Sunday should be a rest day. The week before the event do 10 kilometres (6 miles) on Monday and then from Tuesday to Friday run 5–8 kilometres (3-5 miles) each day, all at a very easy pace. On Saturday go for a very easy 1-kilometre (1000 yards) warm up run and then do two to three stride outs (i.e. pick up the pace and stride out for 20–25 metres (25-30 yards), slow down run slowly for 20–25 metres (25-30 yards) and then do another stride out). Finish with an easy 1-kilometre (1000 yards) warm down. The purpose of the stride outs is to get rid of any residual aches. It is definitely not a speed session.

During the taper don't be tempted to do any heavy training. You will be tempted because of all the hard work you have done over the past three months and you will think about losing fitness. Put these thoughts out of your mind and focus on arriving at the start line feeling fresh. You will not lose fitness during the taper period and any training you do in that period will make no difference to your marathon result. Likewise, if you miss a run during the taper period don't worry it will make no difference to your marathon performance.

Be careful not to overeat during the taper. You have probably increased your food consumption over the previous three months because you needed extra fuel to cope with the increased running. Revert back to your normal pattern of consumption during the taper. In the week before the marathon be sure to drink frequently so that you remain hydrated.

Don't get obsessed with the program. Remember, it's a three-month program (plus taper) and it's the cumulative effect that you are after. Be relaxed if you miss a day and don't try to catch up by doing more the next day.

Appendix 2 – Useful Stretches and Exercises

The calf, quad and hamstring stretches below are the common stretches used by most runners for these muscles. There are many variations and additional exercises for the quads, calf and hamstrings muscles. Each of the exercises below should be repeated two to three times. These stretches should be done before and after each run (before the run to help with the warm up and prepare you mentally, especially for the long run).

Calf stretch

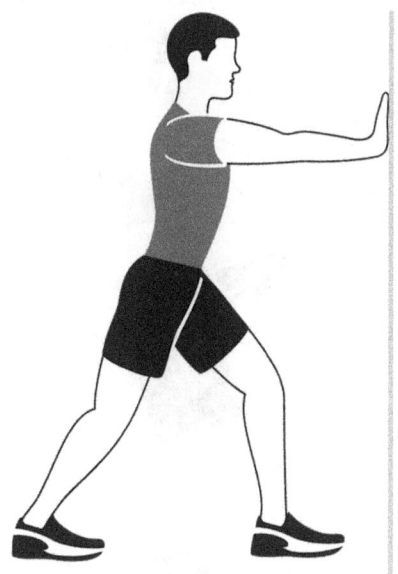

- Stand a little less than arm's distance from the wall.
- Step your left leg forward and your right leg back, keeping your feet parallel.
- Bend your left knee and press through your right heel.
- The back leg must be kept straight with heel on the ground.
- Hold for 30 seconds and switch legs.
- This stretch focuses on the large calf muscle.

Quad stretch

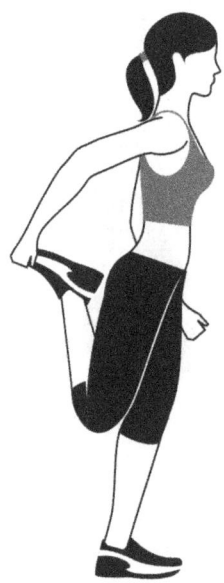

- Stand on your left foot and grab your right shin behind you (hold on to a wall or chair if you need to – doing the stretch without holding on is good for improving balance).
- Tuck your pelvis in, pull your shin towards your glutes (backside), making sure your knee is pointing to the ground.
- Hold for 30 seconds and then switch sides.

Hamstring stretch

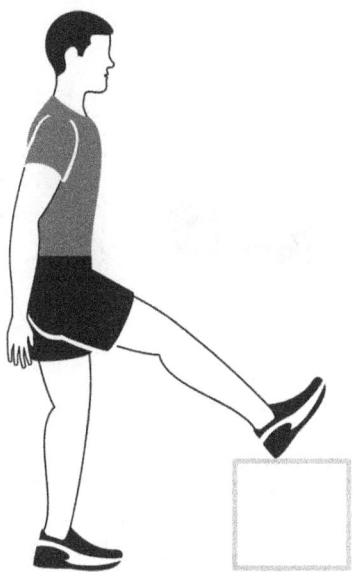

- Prop your left heel up on a surface that is a little lower than your hip, such as a chair or bench.
- Flex your foot. To increase the stretch bend forward towards your flexed foot, by creasing at your hips.
- Some runners find it more effective when they place both hands on the leg that's being stretched.
- Hold for 30 seconds and switch legs.

The plank

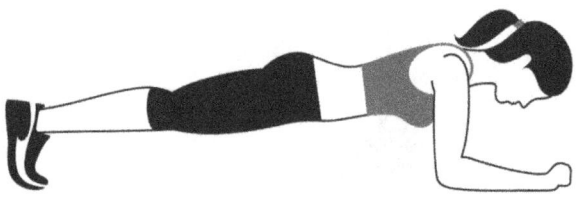

- Start by getting into a push up position. Bend your elbows and rest your weight on your forearms and not on your hands. Your body should form a straight line from shoulders to ankles. Engage your core by sucking your belly button into your spine. Your goal should be to hold it for two minutes. Do this exercise three to four times a week.
- Once you are proficient at planking you might like to try one of the planking variations, which increase the degree of difficulty.

Some Further Reading

The following publications may provide you with inspiration and information about marathons and marathon running.

Bryant, John. 3:59.4. *The Quest to Break the 4 Minute Mile.* Arrow Books 2005.

> Although not about marathon running this is an inspirational tale about determination to achieve a running goal.

Fixx, James F. *The Complete Book of Running.* Outback Press 1978.

> Although a few years old this book is still worth reading. It was the definitive book on running for many years and inspired many people to run and to run marathons.

Gynn, Roger. *The Guinness Book of the Marathon.* Guinness Superlatives Ltd, London 1984.

> This book contains an enormous amount of information about marathons, including history, statistics and many stories about marathon runners.

Henderson, Terry. *See How We Run*. Henderson and Associates Pty Ltd 2000.

>This book is a runners' view of 12 of the great marathons around the world (Sydney, New York, Paris, Vancouver, Rome, Cape Town, San Francisco, Auckland, London, Hong Kong, Chicago and Melbourne).

Howley, Peter. Steve Moneghetti, *In the Long Run. The Making of a Marathon Runner.* Penguin 1996.

>This is the story about Steve Moneghetti, who was ranked as one of the world's best marathon and half marathon runners. The book looks at what motivated him to run a marathon, including what made him stretch his mind and body in one of athletics' most gruelling events.

Hunter, Bob. *The Game's Afoot.* Copyright Publishing Company Pty Ltd 1991.

>This book explores why vigorous exercise is not just essential for physical but also emotional and mental well-being.

Runners World. Sole Motive Pty Ltd. Published monthly.

> This magazine is excellent as it provides a range of tips and other information for runners, including training programs, diet and food information, assessment and reports on events, latest scientific findings, stretching and cross training information, running gear assessment and evaluation of shoes.[3]

Treadwell, Sandy. *The World of Marathons.* Stewart, Tabori & Chang Inc 1987.

> This book captures the details (joys, agonies, determination and triumph of the marathon) by looking in detail at 26 of the iconic marathons around the world. The description is complemented with 165 colour photographs. It also contains a useful pace chart for each 5-kilometre split with finishing times from 2:02:22 to 5:01:24.

---

[3]. Note: An article about 5 runners including the author, entitled *Ageing Racefully,* by Julia Thorn appeared in the August 2006 edition of *Runners World* (pp. 37–43).